Dream Big Trust God

This Journal Belongs To:

_____

Be Still
Stop fighting battles that were not meant for you and see God move on your behalf.

Fresh Manna
Stewanda R. Randolph

What will carry you through?

In the days ahead, what will carry you through?
Will you rely on faith or fear
Will you count on wishes or dreams
Will you hold on to hope or just wait and see what happens?
Will you remain joyful or remember all the things that brought you pain?
We have choices
We can choose how and what we see before us, remaining optimistic or pessimistic
Even in isolation, we can still find ways to gather and socialize
We can choose to keep connections strong, lifting one another up in tough times to help keep faith, hope, joy, and dreams alive and strong.
God has given us the power of innovation, creative ways, and accomplishing much on this earth.
During this time of uncertainty, it is interesting how so many have rediscovered talents they have allowed to go dormant.
Gifts they have dusted off to help create change in the lives of others.
Look at all the new tutorials popping up. We are sharing our gifts to uplift each other, shifting from using them only to gain wealth.
Some have now rediscovered how their God-given gifts, when used properly, can change the life of another, bringing hope, joy, faith, and when this happens, the giver of the gift blesses the one who has used it wisely.
During this time, what will carry you through?
During this time, who will carry you through?
During this time, what will you rely on to get you through?
Will you sit back and rely upon the uncertainty of things to just unfold?
Rediscover the world around you. Find light in disarray as your friends, neighbors, and loved ones rise and blossom, revealing their hidden gifts and sharing with others. Begin to see hope, faith, and joy revealed before your eyes.

Be Still
Stop fighting battles that were not meant for you and see God move on your behalf.

Fresh Manna

Trust in God's love for you and rest in the promises he has for you. Belive that he is God, and will carry you through!

Fresh Manna
Shawanda R. Randolph

Trust in God's love for you and rest in the promises he has for you. Belive that he is God and will carry you through!

Fresh Manna
Shawanda R. Randolph

Trust in God's love for you and rest in the promises he has for you. Belive that he is God, and will carry you through!

Fresh Manna
Shawanda R. Randolph

Be Still
Stop fighting battles that were not meant for you and see God move on your behalf.

Trust in God's love for you and rest in the promises he has for you Belive that he is God, and will carry you through!

Fresh Manna
Shawanda R. Randolph

Trust in God's love for you and rest in the promises he has for you. Belive that he is God, and will carry you through!

Fresh Manna
Shawanda R. Randolph

Trust in God's love for you and rest in the promises he has for you. Belive that he is God and will carry you through!

Fresh Manna
Shawanda R. Randolph

*How do you believe?
Do you put faith in to action
or
pray and wish for things to
come true?*

Fresh Manna
Shawanda R. Randolph

Trust in God's love for you and rest in the promises he has for you. Belive that he is God and will carry you through!

Fresh Manna
Shawanda R. Randolph

Trust in God's love for you and rest in the promises he has for you. Belive that he is God, and will carry you through!

Fresh Manna
Shawanda R. Randolph

www.ingramcontent.com/pod-product-compliance
Lightning Source LLC
Chambersburg PA
CBHW071251070526
44583CB00017B/2421